SUPREMELY

BEING

DEMYSTIFYING THE DEEP CLEANSING PROCESS

Sara Abbas

2017

DISCLAIMER: It should be said that the contents of this book are not intended to treat, cure or prevent any disease or illness. This book details a personal journey through the deep cleansing process and should not be considered "medical advice."

The brand names and products mentioned are in no way affiliated with this publication.

The writer is not in any way affiliated with any product or brand presented.

Any/all endorsements are unsolicited.

Published by: **Ev0lver, Inc.** (Full-Service Talent & Literary Agency)
Ev0lverInc.com
611 K Street, Suite B, #414
San Diego, CA 92101

At the intersection of ancient wisdom and modern science lies an extraordinary world of wellness. Join me as I explore how connecting the best of both worlds can help you achieve better overall health, accelerate your metabolism, balance your hormones, elevate your consciousness, and lose weight *fast* through deep internal cleansing and the magical powers of whole raw foods.

www.SupremelyBeing.com

Dedication

This book is dedicated to the human body. My body, your body, and *every* body was meant to *thrive*. Honor your body, and you will be richly rewarded with the wealth of better health.

Foreword

We live in a world much different than that of our ancestors of even one hundred years ago. Many of us are exposed to industrial chemicals (cleaning products, plasticizers, and cosmetics), air pollution, and tainted water on a daily basis. We consume pharmaceuticals, over-the-counter medications, and food additives, and now more than ever before live hectic lifestyles (stress).

The reality is our world is *full* of toxins and under some conditions, our bodies even *generate* them. The stress we endure can stimulate the release of hormones that contribute to the formation of what are loosely termed prooxidants (reactive oxygen species) and in turn, we consume antioxidants (i.e., vitamin C) to hopefully counteract this imbalance. Stress or "oxidative stress response" also impacts digestion of the foods we consume, as well as the metabolism of endogenous hormones (i.e., estrogen and testosterone) that regulate our homeostasis. Additionally, these stress factors also impact the metabolism of pharmaceuticals and herbal supplements many of us consume along with the absorption of nutrients.

Thankfully, the human body is very forgiving and allows us to heal naturally through detoxification. Detoxification can be bolstered through a deep internal cleanse of the body and its intestinal system, which, in many situations, provides the mind and body a major boost. Cleansing is not just for those with less than perfect eating habits, those under copious amounts of stress, or those at risk for disease. It is not uncommon for someone to consider cleansing following unhealthy eating or on the heels of learning some troubling health news. Indeed, both are terrific reasons to opt for a system detox or to hit your gastrointestinal "reset" button. But one need not endure something abnormal to embrace a deep internal cleanse; it can become a normal part of your life and is not complicated.

The concept of cleansing is not new; our ancestors have been doing variations of cleanses for centuries. Consider that anything with a filter needs cleaning every so often to function optimally (your vehicle's oil and air filters, your drain, etc.). The purification process can result in a wealth of benefits, such as sharpened senses, better absorption of nutrients, improved nerve conduction, and (everyone's favorite) a long-term solution to obesity. As far as the human body is concerned, nothing kick-starts greatness quite like a "clean" slate! For those serious about making drastic changes in their health and living a more *supreme* life, deep cleansing is a sensational place to start.

I hope you are able to use some of the advice, methods, and concepts put forth in these pages. Sara has done a good job of making cleansing understandable.

Sincerely,
Kyle Kramer, Ph.D.

Introduction

Our bodies are incredible machines. Think about all the wonderful things our bodies enable us to do. Be mindful of all your body is doing for you right now; things you never have to even think about like healing, blinking, and filtering toxins from your environment so we can enjoy each and every breath. Our magnificent bodies are constantly repairing, rebuilding, and even regenerating from the inside out. These bodies are capable of handling almost any illness and they house the very energy that creates life itself. Talk about significant!

With that in mind, I intended to start fresh on my journey to overall wellness via deep cleansing. I wanted to press the "Reset" button, detoxify my entire body, to allow it to fully heal, function, and thrive as intended. With improved health, also came a leaner, sexier physique, as a healthy digestive system and "clean" eating allows for optimal metabolizing and energy conversion.

WARNING: Deep Cleansing is not for quitters. While anyone can have sensational results with just a raw diet alone, truly deep cleansing requires some dedication, a little will power, and (most importantly) trust. A positive outlook and open mind will serve you well if you choose to embark upon a similar journey. Without exaggeration, your results can be miraculous if you respect the process, understand the "why" behind the explored techniques, and use your best instincts (trust your gut) to create an experience that is best for *your* body.

Table of Contents

Chapter One
General Overview on Cleansing

Somehow, the innocent topic of cleansing has become a very touchy subject. Nearly all who have committed themselves to one sort of cleanse or another can get a little defensive about his/her method being *the best* (consider "my baby is the cutest, my religion is the rightist," etc.).

The truth? *Everyone* **is correct**.

The inner workings of our bodies and digestive tracts are as individual as our thumbprints, so everyone has different needs that can be met via different diets and different cleansing methods. With all that is out there, it can be difficult to discern which one of these many methods is worthy of *your* precious time, so I'm going to assist with that process...

Evaluate your goals beforehand. Deciding what you want out of a cleanse can help narrow down the options. Take a tip from Stephen Covey and "Begin with the End in Mind."

Chapter Two
Top 5 Most Common Cleanse Goals

1)   **General Detox:** Some simply want to live healthier lifestyles or to kick-start healthier habits. Ridding your digestive tract of basic surface toxins can be a phenomenal boost for the immune system and major organs of the body, among other benefits. To reap more rewards of your current health/fitness regimens, a deep detoxifying cleanse may be right for you.

2)   **Weight Loss**: There are a number of ways cleansing can result in weight loss. The most significant is the fact that cleansing the digestive tract can lead to more efficient digestion and a speedy metabolism. The marvelous thing about a "deep cleanse" is that the weight loss can easily be sustained as long as the body stays on the right track with the right "clean" foods and one does not "re-pollute" the system with toxins (additives, preservatives, and chemicals); some of these will be unavoidable but making a conscious effort can and will change your life. Also, any drastic reduction in caloric intake (as experienced with most deep cleanses) will most likely result in lost weight.

3)   **Addressing an Illness or Health Concern**: It's no secret that deep cleansing has been known to aid in the improvement of health issues such as high cholesterol, diabetes, heart problems, intestinal blockages, asthma, allergies, endocrine issues, thyroid inactivity, acne, depression, migraines, cancers, hormonal imbalances, and *much* more. For those seeking a clean slate health-wise, a deep cleanse can be a literal lifesaver.

4)   Emotional Healing: Recent studies have shown there is much to be said about that "gut feeling" of yours. Mainstream science is now beginning to support the idea that emotions can be stored in the digestive tract, particularly the intestines. There has been a longstanding belief in Indian Ayurveda as well as Chinese reflexology, among other ancient wellness institutions. Purification rituals, such as deep cleansing, can provide a means for releasing those stored emotions, thus enabling us to overcome them and move into higher levels of consciousness.

5)   Addiction Cessation: Being mindful of your consumption habits as related to food can greatly improve your ability to overcome addictive tendencies. Every one of us is able to master what we choose to eat; unless Mom is still packing you a lunch, you probably choose what you want (in

one way or another) each and every day! Cleansing can boost your confidence in self-mastery and help you regain control in *any* area of your life.

Chapter Three
Common Methods of Effective "Deep" Cleansing

With all the info out there, it can be an overwhelming process, not to mention difficult, to discern what will be best for your body. Consider the following before exploring my process.

RAW Plant-based Diets: These are especially beneficial for those who eat any amount of red meat or consume a high percentage of animal proteins (including poultry, milk/dairy/whey, pork, etc.). Taking some time to allow the body to operate on raw, unprocessed, uncooked fruits and vegetables is a rewarding, vibrant way of cleansing, especially for those who may not be physically or psychologically ready for a juice cleanse.

Juicing: The term "juicing" in this context refers to simply consuming only juices, no solid foods. There is plenty of controversy about juicing alone. I've personally thrived for over three weeks on juice alone and know many others who have done it longer. It can be perfectly safe for those in good health. But, like anything else, if you are not prepared emotionally or are not well enough physically to "juice" – then don't! Honor your body. It's that simple. If you are feeling well and are seeking to deeply cleanse, you can surely see incredible results in as little as 36 hours of straight juicing.

Fasting: By fasting I mean zero solid food whatsoever, and no juice or other liquids, only water. This is an especially controversial option. Any medical professional (Eastern, Western, or otherwise) will advise to do this very cautiously (or more likely, not to do it at all). The truth is, unless you're raking sand in a Tibetan monastery, you'll probably have to function in society, and will want to maintain your usual physical and cognitive functionality. Water alone, while it won't *kill* you (at least not for a while), can reduce your strength, slow down your thought process, and inhibit your ability to keep up with a demanding schedule. So, to remedy this and do it safely (without setting you back professionally), you can supplement a water fast with liquid minerals and herbs to ensure you're getting what you need without consuming food or even juice. A high-quality greens supplement throughout the day (I like Green Vibrance), trace minerals (I like Source Naturals Colloidal Trace Minerals), and various immune boosting herbal extracts (such as Astragalus, Myrrh, Echinacea, etc.) are great ways to ensure you stay healthy for your fast, if you choose to go that route. I'll elaborate on the benefits of the aforementioned herbs later in the "ingredients" section.

But, with many paths up the mountain comes many methods to achieving Deep Cleansing success…

Chapter Four
The Breakdown

After nearly 12 years of reading, researching, and old-fashioned trial and error experimentation, I discovered a precise amalgamation of methods that really worked for me and changed my life in ways I simply cannot begin to list. I found *my* success in a carefully combined regimen of raw food, juicing, and fasting (together), which I will further detail very soon. This method has worked wonders for others in my life as well. Nearly all who are close to me have incorporated some, if not all of these techniques into their lives and 100% have seen improvement.

For those who know me, I make no secret of the fact that cleansing has paved my way to incredible health; having practically grown up in hospitals, it's hard to imagine that I haven't taken (or needed) a prescription in years. Ailments and challenges of mine such as asthma, allergies, years of hypothyroidism, hormonal imbalances, and other chronic issues began to disappear after embarking on my journey to better overall health. At the end of all this experimenting, I'm still learning more and more about the body every day. But, it brings me immense joy to share with you the findings of *my* journey to pressing the "Reset" button for my health, once and for all.

Chapter Five
Introducing The *Supremely Being* Hybrid Cleanse; *The* Cleanse; The Best of Deep Cleansing in One!

Desperate to free myself from the trappings of life-long medical conditions, I tried *everything*. Juice cleanses, grapefruit cleanses, various Master Cleanses, lemon-maple syrup-pepper cleanses, oil pulling regimens, clay-based detox cleanses, liquid diets, high-carbs/low-carb detox diets, gluten-free, paleo, dairy-free, vegan, pescatarian, elimination diets of all sorts, and *much* more. You name it – I tried it all. Many made me thinner, in one way or another. And, nearly everything I tried had, at least, some small benefit.

Something nearly all cleanses had in common was the elimination of notoriously "bad" things from your routine while partaking in them; the usual suspects such as cigarettes, alcohol (even wine/beer), and processed foods where nowhere to be found in any of the truly effective methods. And, it should come as no surprise that <u>you will indeed have to eliminate them if you intend to see results from this sort of deep cleanse</u> as well.

Something also important to note at this time is the fact that there are many beneficial cleanses out there that are much less intense. This is, in no way, distracting from the benefits of the aforementioned methods. However, once the digestive tract is deeply cleansed, the body is better enabled to reap the benefits of the other methods.

Why is deep cleansing so important? There are much more technical and precise ways of explaining this, but I'm going to break it down in a simple way that helps me remember to eat right always, not just when I'm cleansing…

Our bodies have to process not only what we ingest, but also what we are physically exposed to. Chemicals in the air, unnatural ingredients or preservatives in packaged or processed foods, toxins from old illnesses, buildup of lactic acid and chemicals caused by injuries, harmful substances in lotions or beauty products, etc. All of these things pass through our system in one way or another, eventually making their way to our digestive tract (either through consumption or absorption). Raw, natural foods are easily processed and waste is created in a very simple manner. However, when it comes to the other aforementioned items, much is *not* processed by the body, and can remain inside your system, typically being stored in the intestinal walls. An indulgent meal here or there will not hurt you, but think back to before we had the access to the health resources we have now. If you had unhealthy habits, say – perhaps in college, the effects of the damage to your body can still be present inside you, in the lining of your intestines. Fast foods, trans fats, highly acidic compounds, all sorts of things can be stored on the intestinal walls. Over just a short period of time, the entire intestinal tract can become coated with stored pockets of all this unprocessed "junk." Layer upon layer, week after week, (not to mention) year after year, and you've completely coated the lining of your intestines. Yuck. But so what? Well, the walls of your intestines are where nutrients are extracted from the foods you eat, for one. So by having all this "junk" built up inside your intestines, you are severely limiting your body's ability to extract vital nutrients from what you consume, causing vitamin deficiencies, unnecessary hunger, lethargy, and a bevy of other metabolic and general health issues.

Can't I just begin making healthier choices now, and avoid cleansing altogether? Making healthier choices is a great start, but it's not quite that simple. Imagine you have a very dirty fish tank, full of toxic bacteria and algae. You don't

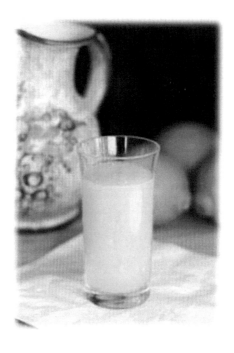

want your precious fish to get sick and die, so you have to clean the tank. Simple. But, you don't *clean* the tank just by adding clean water. That only creates more dirty water! The same principle applies to your body. You don't press the "reset" button on your health by simply eating more salads. <u>You have to cut out the bad and actually "clean the tank.</u>" *Then* when you incorporate those healthy new habits into your lifestyle, they will make a significant impact.

Chapter Six
Benefits of Deep Cleansing

Absorption of Nutrients: Without properly cleaning the layers of "junk" from the intestinal lining, you will not be able to really feel the nutrients from your food.

Before I cleansed, I absolutely never felt energized from things like spinach or leafy vegetables. I never felt full or satisfied from fruits and vegetables alone. I never felt anything but hungry until I deeply cleansed the intestinal tract.

All the great detox/cleanse methods out there like herbal teas, juice diets, water fasting and enzymes in the world cannot remove that intestinal "junk" quite like a total intestinal cleanse.

Shrinking of the Gut: As you can imagine, these layers of toxicity and pockets of inflammation can cause the intestines to enlarge. In many cases, this is the reason for a protruding gut, especially on those who may be otherwise thin.

As you eliminate the toxins from your system and reduce inflammation, many will notice a significant decrease in the size of their gut. Some major causes of inflammation are typically highly acidic foods/substances (alcohol, nicotine, wheat, processed sugars, etc.). By "cleaning the tank" and eliminating these items from your routine, you can quite literally shrink your gut and keep it slim.

For those who are already physically fit, a good deep cleanse can help pave the way for seeing results you may be missing with exercise alone. When resuming your physical fitness routine after a deep cleanse, many find it easier to achieve results and see well-defined abdominal muscles where they were not visible before.

Increased Bowel Activity: This may not be a very glamorous benefit, but it sure is a sign of great health! Many who have high levels of toxicity in their bodies experience only one bowel movement per day.

But, think back to when we were babies, before the toxicity, before the preservatives, before we had time to soil our innards with unhealthy foods and habits. Most babies have bowel movements after each meal, or about three times per day. Of course it will take more time for food to move through an adult intestinal tract, but the concept is clear – less toxicity, more efficiency. Heathy bowel movements are a sign of an efficient system.

After you've effectively deep cleansed the intestinal tract, food will move through much more quickly (especially if you are eating "clean" raw foods), and you can expect more frequent bowel movements. This is a fantastic sign that your body is metabolizing efficiently and helps ensure the health of your kidneys and colon as well.

Permanent Weight Loss: Going back to the "absorption of nutrients" benefit above, when your body is not able to properly extract the nutrients from the food you eat, they essentially become empty calories. Your body isn't able to "use" much off this food, so your food's purpose is basically only to satisfy cravings and habitual needs. Then, much of what is not processed out right away is stored in the body as tissue.

However, after a successful deep cleanse, the body is able to properly metabolize what you consume, leading to weight loss. You'll find that this weight stays off as long as you maintain healthy habits moving forward too, that's the beauty of it. It's not like water-weight that goes right back on, it's gone for good!

Improved Function of the Nervous System: All of these toxins we've discussed interfere with our senses in one way or another. Some cause pains, migraines, unexplained aches here or there, shortness of breath, soreness, gas, bloating, and a number of other common physical ailments.

When we nurture our precious bodies, and properly cleanse the digestive tract, these issues often disappear. Many will also experience noticeable improvements in areas such as vision, reflexes, memory, and more prominent instincts or intuition (more noticeable "gut feelings"). Other negatives such as anxiety and stress will often disappear as the body is better able to balance itself chemically.

More Energy: This is a huge one. So many people ask, "Well, if you're just drinking juice, aren't you tired all the time?" This couldn't be further from reality. The fact is, the more processed and complex our food is, the harder our bodies have to work to break that down. With packaged processed foods, preservatives, cooking oils, etc. our bodies have to work extra hard to break it all down so we can digest it. If you're consuming a big juicy steak, for instance, think about how difficult that is just to chew, then imagine your body having to further break that down just to get it through your system. Now, compare *that* to drinking a juice; you just drink it and boom- ready to digest! Your body doesn't have to put as much effort into breaking it down, so you'll feel more energized because less effort is being exerted. This is the same reason we can feel sluggish after a big meal or after eating dense, "heavy" foods. The less work your body has to do, the more energy you will have. So why not simply choose healthy options that are easy for your body to digest, like whole raw foods or juices, and give yourself the gift of abundant energy?

Ridding the Body of Major Sources of Most Diseases:
The gut is the epicenter of disease in the body. Many believe that the source of most illness and disease stem from bacteria and toxicity stored in the gut. It only makes sense, that when the gut is truly clean, it can no longer harbor disease. Going back to the concept of 'making life easier on your body,' when you choose the right raw foods and juices that are easy to digest, your body is not having to devote as much energy to digestion; believe it or not, digestion can be a *completely* exhausting process for the body, especially for someone with a compromised immune system or serious illness.

When the body does not have to deal with breaking down what we are eating or the chemicals we are putting on our skin and hair, when we are able to live our lives in a reasonably toxic-free manner, then (and only then), the body can begin to do what it's supposed to do and address any illnesses, injuries or disease. Our cells are constantly repairing, regenerating, and curing from the inside out. These abilities are amplified in ways one simply cannot describe when we are free of toxins. Our bodies are incredibly powerful self-healing mechanisms. When we deeply cleanse and then eliminate these toxins from our routine, we allow our bodies the freedom to do what they were meant to do. This ultimately leads to remarkable health.

Chapter Seven
The **Cleanse**

When I discovered that a raw plant-based diet, juicing, and intermittent fasting worked very well for me, I naturally wondered why we couldn't combine them. I soon discovered that others *had,* indeed, combined them, but no one presented it in a way that worked for me. I wanted easy-to-follow, straightforward details, and maximum results in the shortest (but safest) amount of time.

And so, with these thoughts in my back pocket, I developed a supreme combination…

Pre-cleanse Prep: Lasts about 7 days, and suggests consuming 2.5 – 3 meals per day of plant-based foods only to acclimate the body to a raw, plant-based diet.

This week is for acclimating to a raw, plant-based diet that does not include anything that will cause inflammation. These foods to avoid can be found later, but most importantly eliminates gluten, dairy, and meat from one's diet. During this week, there is also a strong emphasis on maintaining high levels of alkalinity to ensure healthy immune function throughout the actual cleanse. Alcohol and other harmful substances should be avoided during all levels of a deep cleanse, so plan accordingly if that is part of your lifestyle on a regular basis.

Cleanse – Level 1: Lasts 7 days and includes a combination of whole, organic detoxifying agents as well as herbs and minerals, and consuming no more than 2 meals per day, of raw, plant-based foods only.

Cleanse – Level 2: Lasts 7 days and includes a combination of whole, organic detoxifying agents as well as herbs and minerals, and consuming no more than 1 meal per day of raw, plant-based foods only.

Cleanse – Level 3: Lasts 7 days and includes a combination of whole, organic detoxifying agents as well as herbs and minerals, and consuming only fresh, organic juice, without solid food.

Post-Cleanse: Lasts 4 – 7 days and includes "clean" eating with minimal solids in order to comfortably ease one's way back into eating more.

A Note on Flexibility: Alternating between Levels may be necessary for someone not seeking to fully dive in just yet. If you have many upcoming social obligations or do not have the will power to drink only liquids for a period of time, then consider skipping Level 3 entirely, or perhaps don't do an entire week. Be gentle with yourself. Or, if you get a few days into Level 3 and the effects of the cleanse are hindering your work in some way or you feel too tired to function properly in your work/ life roles, then (by all means) switch back to Level 2. The cleanse will still prove to be very effective. But, like all great things in life, in order to achieve amazing results, you will have to put in effort to make it happen.

"... be gentle with yourself. You are a child of the universe. No less than the trees and the stars..."

~Max Ehrmann, *Desiderata*

Chapter Eight
What to Eat for Best Results?

The key here was for me to eat foods that were easiest to digest, such as the following:

Almonds (preferably sprouted or soaked)

Apples

Apple cider vinegar, balsamic vinegar

Asparagus

Avocados

Bananas

Beets

Berries (Blueberries, Strawberries, Cherries, etc.)

Broccoli

Cabbage

Carrots

Chia Seeds (preferably sprouted)

Cucumbers

Corn on the cob, (not canned, fresh & raw)

Dates

Dried fruits (no added sugar, not glazed, and not with Sulphur or any additives)

Eggplants

Flax Seeds (preferably sprouted / soaked)

Fresh Fruit Juices

Fresh Veggie Juices

Garlic

Grapefruit

Hemp Seeds

Herbal or Green Teas (caffeine free)

Honey (raw)

Lemon

Lettuce and Greens (dandelion greens, kale, any greens, any lettuce, spinach, etc.)

Maple syrup, organic

Melons

Oil – used sparingly (only the following: avocado oil, coconut oil, flaxseed oil, grapeseed oil, olive oil, saffron oil, sunflower oil, walnut oil)

Oranges

Papayas

Pears

Quinoa (mind your portion sizes)

Radishes

Raisins

Seasoning (fresh or dried herbs are perfectly fine)

Spinach

Sprouts

Superfood Greens (Kelp, Spirulina, Chlorella)

Sweet Potatoes (these may be cooked, but do not eat
more than 2 or 3 times per week)

Tangerines

Vegetables (all fresh vegetables, nothing canned)

Vegetable Broth

Vegetable Soups

Walnuts (preferably sprouted or soaked)

Wheat Grass Juiced

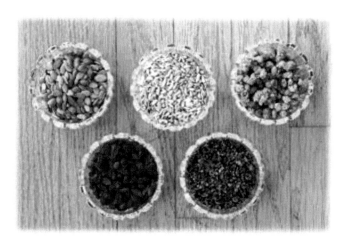

Chapter Nine
What Should Be Avoided While Deep Cleansing?

Alcohol (yes, even beer and wine should be omitted for all levels of deep cleansing)

Animal Proteins (Fish, Meat, Pork, Poultry, Red Meat, Shellfish, etc.)

Barley

Black or white pepper

Bread, baked

Caffeine

Canned or microwaved fruits and vegetables

Carbonated Liquids

Cereals (all of them, anything in a box really can wait for a month)

Chocolate (I know, it's "good for you" but the sugar and dairy ingredients are not conducive to a deep cleanse)

Cigarettes (don't even think about it!)

Coffee (I know... *I know*)

Dairy (all products derived from dairy such as milk, cheese, cream, butter, etc.)

Eggs

Foods cooked with oil

Gluten (see also: wheat)

Grains, except quinoa and millet

Legumes (this includes ALL beans and also peanuts)

Oatmeal

Pasta

Pepper (all kinds)

Popcorn

Preservatives

Processed foods

Salt (including Celtic, sea and Himalayan)

Sodas (any soft drinks really, even soda water)

Soy (tofu, tempeh, etc.)

Sugar (Brown, Processed, White, etc.)

Sweeteners, artificial

Tea (unless caffeine free)

Vinegar (unless apple cider vinegar)

Wheat (any/all forms of it, and anything glutinous)

Chapter Ten
Common Concerns & FAQs

How did you get your protein? I hear this all the time. The truth is, unless you're an athlete by trade, you will get plenty of protein from the eating a variety of healthy foods. Basically, everything except oil contains some amount of protein. Though sometimes small, some amount of protein can be found in broccoli, spinach, cauliflower, soaked/sprouted nuts, avocados, and sprouts especially.

The minerals and vitamins that can actually be absorbed while eating a plant-based diet can be shockingly good. Many report not feeling tired at all, and, in fact, feeling incredibly energized from the "live" raw foods.

If you feel you still need more protein for one reason or another, there are plenty of unprocessed superb plant-based protein powders on the market. I like Life's Basics Hemp Protein.

It's superb mixed with a little almond, flax, or coconut milk (I can't get enough of vanilla almond milk with Life's Basics "Unsweetened Vanilla").

I love cooked food! Can I cheat? Yes. But, only a little. And, only if you absolutely *must* have cooked food. I understand wanting the comfort of a hot meal, so it's okay to have grilled or steamed veggies in Levels 1 and 2, but no frying or microwaving.

How did you survive not eating 2000 calories per day?
This one blows me away because logic alone tells us that 2000
calories per day is <u>not</u> a very good one-size-fits-all idea.

Let's say, for instance, we're talking about a 30-year-old
woman who weighs 130lbs. If she is fairly physically active,
she is probably burning about 1200 – 1600 calories per day.
If she consumes 2000 calories per day, then, clearly, there are
400 – 800 (unburned) calories being stored every day. That is
not even weight maintenance, that is actively gaining weight
every day! And, if you're that 30-year-old woman, I'm sure
you know *exactly* where those calories are being stored too.
Deep cleansing will help open your eyes to how little the
body really needs in terms of calories. It will help you realize
when you reach for certain foods because it's a certain time
of day or perhaps because a certain activity triggers a craving
for something specific.

**Rarely do we reach for food out of actual "hunger."
Typically, when we reach for food, it's just the time
during the day we usually eat, so we do until we break
the cycle with a cleanse or resolution.**

Being mindful of this can make a huge impact on your life
moving forward.

Don't you miss cooked food? In all honesty, eating "live"
raw foods felt so good that after my 3rd deep cleanse, I didn't
go back to cooked food and still eat 90% – 100% raw every
day, with the exception of steamed or cooked vegetables on
rare occasions.

I am continuously overwhelmed with gratitude every morning I wake up feeling wonderful; it's a beautiful thing – especially after years of sickness! The health benefits were undoubtedly drastic, but when I noticed things like my reflexes improve and noticeable improvements in my reaction times, my hearing and even my moods, I didn't *want* to go back to cooked foods! And, there's something amazing about your food being ready to eat the moment you prepare it. Waiting for something to bake or cook is such a bore now.

Natural flavor is in foods stand out more now. Because I'm not consuming a lot of additives and my taste buds are no longer dealing with a bevy of chemicals; the tasting notes in my foods are more pronounced, my senses are keener, and although I love flavorful (sometimes even spicy foods), I no longer feel the need to mask anything with spice or condiments, natural flavors really excite me.

Eating Organic Is Expensive, Can I Cut Corners to Save Some Coin? First off, that's a myth. There are *plenty* of inexpensive organic options, but the key is to shop around for what's *in season* and keep an open mind. For instance, out-of-season organic strawberries may cost a fortune in November, but organic broccoli, kale, cabbage, and a number of awesome root vegetables are in season and won't cost you a bundle.

Make the most of your money and do it the right way, give it 100% if pressing the "Reset" button is important for you. Also, not dining out will save you a bundle because you'll most likely be taking your own food wherever you go and dining at home so you can prepare your own fresh, ray foods.

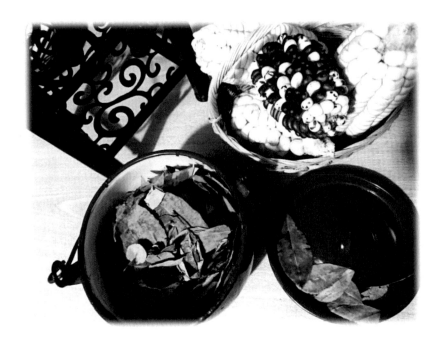

Chapter Eleven
Maximizing Results

In order to get the most from a deep cleanse experience, one should consider the following:

Start Healthy: Do not begin a deep cleanse unless you're in fairly good health. A compromised immune system needs extra nourishment and care to heal before beginning a cleanse. Though wonderful, these can be taxing on the body.

Commit to Change: Unless you fall ill or are physically unable to continue with a regimen, then do your body a favor by committing yourself 100% to any cleanse you choose.

Vegan Products: To amplify the effects of any cleanse, use only plant-based products on your nails, hair, and skin (the largest organ of your body). Switching to plant-based, gluten-free, lotions, shampoos, and make-up (if you must), will drastically improve the benefits of *any* cleanse. Read your labels and look for the organic, non-GMO, vegan symbols on products, or simply make your own. The less chemicals you put on your body, the less you'll have to get rid of when you cleanse. This is also a sensational habit to hang onto if you can stick to it long-term.

My simple rule of thumb is: if I wouldn't put it in my mouth, then I won't put it on my skin!

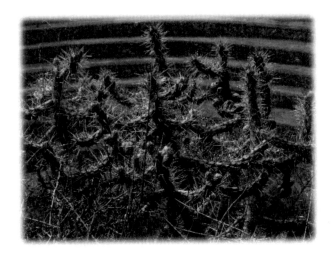

Pre-Cleanse Diet: Don't skip this step, it's nearly as important as the cleanse itself. The pre-cleanse week is one for paving the way to more mindful dining, clearing out the tempting food (if you don't trust yourself to behave later in the cleanse), and getting your ingredients together so you are ready to cleanse. Get as hydrated as you can and load up on electrolytes so you are well-stocked for the rewarding journey ahead.

Organic Food: As tempting as it may be, eating conventionally grown foods will only slow down the cleanse process and keep you from getting the results you want. While they may not "hurt" you in ways you notice right away, it will be one more layer of toxins your body has to get rid of before it can begin its health and wellness mission.

Food Prep: Some cleansers cheat themselves out of the deepest (and most effective) levels of cleansing by eating non-recommended foods out of sheer of convenience. Don't let

that be your excuse, you deserve amazing results! Pay it
forward with food prep, and you'll *always* have something
healthy available when meal or juice time rolls around. I like
to set aside a little time on the weekends to clean, peel and
chop veggies and make or purchase juices. Store the fruits
and veggies in Tupperware or single-serving baggies for
taking to work or wherever you go that may not have fresh
fruit and veggies.

> **Tip**: lining containers and baggies with parchment paper
> before filling with vegetables will help keep them fresh
> and crisp longer.

Honor Your Body: Most cleanses or dietary changes can be
especially challenging on the 2nd or 3rd day of juicing (in my
case, Day 2 and 3 of Level 3), once you make it past that little
hump, however, the rest is easy – promise! It's typical to feel
very quick, mild symptoms arise as you rid yourself of toxins
that cause bacterial infections (quick headaches, brief
soreness of muscles or throat, slight soreness of old injuries,
etc.). The less our body has to focus on breaking down
complex food, the more it can focus on healing old injuries
and ridding itself of harmful toxins. These "mild" symptoms
are typically just a sign that your body is finally able to heal
these things once and for all – get excited! However, do pay
attention to the cues of your body. If something is deeply
painful, or if you begin to feel really sick for any length of
time, stop the cleanse. Your body may not be ready for that
sort of intensity just yet. And that's okay.

Chapter Twelve
The Secret Sauce: Proper Food Combining

Different foods digest at different speeds, this is nothing new. There is an entire area of science dedicated to the study of food combining called Trophology; if you want a healthy, *speedy* metabolism, the studies basically suggest that foods should only be combined when they digest at a similar speed. This also ensures that you get the most nutrients out of what you eat. Even if you're eating relatively "clean," careless combinations can lead to a slower metabolism, as well as a bevy of digestive complications, here's why…

Imagine you have a plain baked potato, followed by a bowl of berries. Seems like a harmless, healthy lunch, right? Think just a moment about the foods themselves though; berries are mostly water, so if you had eaten those first (and waited about 30 – 40 minutes before eating anything else) they would be fully digested and all of those nutrients and antioxidants would be in your system. However, when they are eaten after a starchy vegetable, like a baked potato, they have to hang out and wait to be digested. **Starchy carbohydrates can take 3 – 12 hours to be digested, all the while those little berries are in your digestive tract, waiting impatiently. The acidity created by all this waiting around causes fermentation, which <u>translates to you experiencing bloating or gas</u>.** Meanwhile, your body is still trying to break that potato down and use it, but ends up converting much of it into fat because there's a fermented ruckus to tend to on the horizon. At the end of it all, you've cheated yourself out of the energy and fulfillment of the starch as well as the nutrients of the berries.

Not to say you *have* to wait between foods all the time, but being mindful of this concept can work wonders for your metabolism. **Simply put, eating water-rich roods first and denser ones later will make a big difference**. Here are some other food combining tips and a helpful chart to help you on this journey.

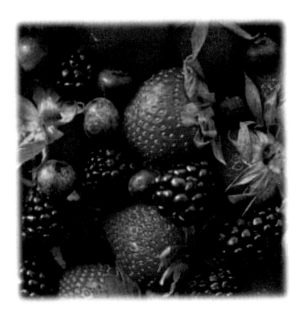

Chapter Thirteen
Food Combining Facts

1) Melons digest extremely quickly, so these are best eaten alone.

2) Foods are *much* easier to digest when they are already broken down for the body (blended or preferably juiced).

3) Greens are super outgoing and get along well with pretty much all foods.

4) It's easier for your body to digest one thing at a time, so be gentle (this is one of the many reasons I avoid meat).

5) Stay hydrated and drink plenty of water 15 – 20 minutes before your meal, but try not to drink much *during* meals, if convenient – wait a little while (30 – 60 minutes) for your food to be digested *before* "washing it down."

6) Do not combine fruits with vegetables. Period. Unless we're talking about greens, leafy greens and lettuce may be combined with anything.

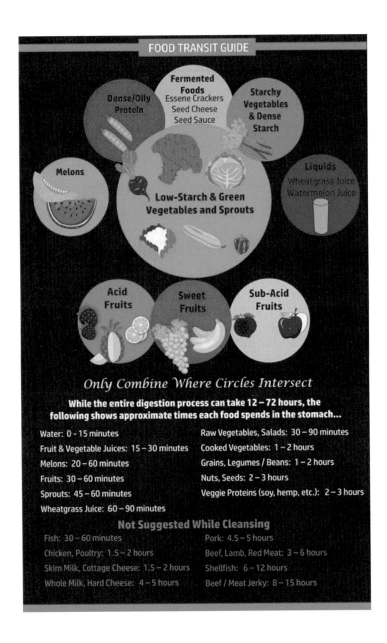

Chapter Fourteen
The Ingredients for Better Health

Liquids Are Best: When possible, I try to choose supplements in liquid extract form over pills because they are easier to digest and the bioavailability is typically far more potent than most in capsule or pill form. When your body does not have to worry about breaking down a gel-cap, it can immediately begin extracting nutrients from the supplement. Liquids will be in your system quicker and are much easier for your body to use. For this reason, some liquid extracts may cost a little more than their competitors, simply because you *typically* get more nutrients from a liquid or powder product (even when the amounts are the same). There are exceptions to this, of course. So, do your homework and read your labels.

Clean, High-Quality Ingredients: One should also be mindful of organic/non-GMO supplements. Psyllium, for instance, is an excellent fiber and can play a vital role in the deep cleansing process. However, some conventionally grown psylliums can do more harm than good as chemicals and toxifying agents are easily carried within the many crevices of this grain's husks (much like corn, *always* make sure your corn is organic/non-GMO). Look for a high-quality product with Organic and non-GMO labels as often as possible.

Necessary and Optional Ingredients: Not all of these will be necessary for a deep cleanse ("necessary" ingredients will be noted as will "optional"), but before beginning any detox program, read your labels. Some of these you may want to continue on a regular basis. Astragalus, for instance, is an excellent immune-booster and I still take it every day. Some of these ingredients can be found in the same supplement, I've noted that at the bottom with asterisks, do yourself a favor and avoid having to find these individually by getting

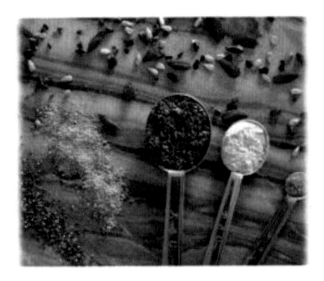

the suggested compound. Many of these have far too many benefits to list, so here's a quick summary of why you may want to incorporate them into *your* cleanse...

Chapter Fifteen
My Necessary Ingredients

Vitamin B 12 (liquid): This is a fantastic way to feel energized and elevate your mood while the body undergoes any sort of changes, like a deep cleanse. If you are getting some B-12 in a multivitamin already, you are most likely not getting enough to notice the effects.

Many natural/plant-based vitamin B12 products are derived from Beetroot, like the one mentioned below. The healers of ancient Rome used Beetroot as a treatment for fevers and constipation. They made soups and stews to get higher concentrations of Beetroot nutrients into their patient's digestive systems quickly and conveniently, not unlike modern juicing.

We now have more streamlined methods of getting natural B12 these days. I really like the Garden of Life – MyKind Organics B-12 Organic Spray; this Vegan product is simply sprayed in your mouth and is made entirely of organic, whole foods. I took about 500 mcgs three times daily throughout my cleanse. There are many options out there for B12, but I was careful only to choose plant-based supplements for optimal cleansing.

Bentonite: This will be a key detox component of your cleanse and it *must* be in liquid form. Bentonite is like a magnet for heavy metals and toxins in your system, when used properly for a short amount of time (less than a month), it can be an incredibly powerful means of total body detoxification.

I like Great Plains Liquid Bentonite because it has a high concentration of the active component, montmorillonite, which is a superb binding agent. I took 1 tablespoon three times daily, mixed with Psyllium and 10 oz of distilled water. Learn more about that in the Planner.

Cascara Sagrada Bark*: This exciting substance was a favorite of the Native Americans for aiding in digestive healing. The bark comes in concentrated extract form and stimulates the adrenal glands as well as gall bladder to increase secretions in the stomach, liver, and pancreas for optimal digestion.

I like Nature's Secret – Super Cleanse Tablets, which includes this and a number of other ingredients on this list, noted with one asterisk. I took one tablet three times daily during my cleanse, as directed.

Cayenne*: Cayenne is a powerful stimulant that greatly assists in the cleansing and rebuilding of digestive tissue during the deep cleansing process. It also increases the effectiveness of other herbs.

I like Nature's Secret – Super Cleanse Tablets (mentioned above), which includes this and a number of other ingredients on this list, noted with one asterisk. I took one tablet three times daily, as directed, during my cleanse. Herb Pharm also makes a great cayenne extract in liquid form.

Chebulic Myrobalan* (fruit in powder or extract form, aka: Haritaki, Harad or Haleelaz): This mystical herb comes in seven varieties and each is known to have immense healing powers. The Vijaya variety is considered the most potent, predominantly found in Northern India, but can be found in markets of the Near and Far East. According to ancient Ayurvedic scripts, healers used this to aid in the treatment of a number of diseases and it is commonly known to assist digestion, regulate acidity, and address bacterial issues caused by food poisoning. Its cleansing properties are impressive and even a small amount can make a big difference in a deep cleanse.

This is a little harder to find outside of India and the Middle East. The dried fruit is readily available online, but then it must be ground into a fine powder for digestion. I took one half teaspoon (just under 3 grams) twice daily during my cleanse, mixing it with my Greens and Maca. For an easier means of getting it, Nature's Secret – Super Cleanse Tablets (mentioned above), actually includes this in their formula, and a number of other ingredients on this list, noted with one asterisk.

Vitamin D (liquid): Vitamin D works wonders for the immune system and studies show we almost never get enough naturally. Also, recommended daily values have been grossly underestimated for years, so supplementing this during a cleans (and even after) is a good idea. Vitamin D is a crucial part of maintaining healthy immune function.

I like Garden of Life – MyKind Organics D3 Organic Spray; this vegan product is sprayed in your mouth, is made entirely of organic, whole foods, and it contains a heaping side of healthy Omegas! I did one spray twice daily, as directed, during my cleanse.

Dandelion Root: This vitamin-rich, multi-tasking blood purifier helps cleanse the liver and can aide in hypoglycemia, gall bladder, spleen, and a number of stomach problems. The name of its Genus, Taraxacum, is thought to be derived from the Greek word "taraxo" (meaning disorder) and "akos" (meaning remedy), on account of the many medicinal uses for this underrated plant. Dried or boiled dandelion root was a go-to Native American remedy for a number of digestive issues, kidney disease, swelling, skin problems, and much more.   There are countless studies shown to prove its powerful effects on liver detoxification, especially, so I made it a necessity during my deep cleanses and continue to take it daily long after the cleanses.

Dandelion Root is readily available, and can be found in virtually *any* health food store or supplement shop. I like Herb Pharm Dandelion herbal extract. I took one full dropper (about 807 mg or .7 ml) three times daily during my cleanse.

Goldenseal**:   This underrated herb helps improve liver functionality, and clear impurities from the bronchial pathways as well as the throat, intestines, stomach, and bladder. The Cherokee people used Goldenseal to treat cancer and treat local infections, among other important uses. Goldenseal is considered a rare "active responder" sometimes used as an herbal antibiotic and considered a useful tool in the treatment of digestive inflammation.

I found that Herb Pharm's Echinacea Goldenseal compound extract effectively combined both herbs in one formula. I took one full dropper (about .7 ml or roughly 646 mg of the blended extract) three times daily during my cleanse.

Greens (superfood powder)***: One of the most important components of a deep cleanse, a stellar high-quality "greens" compound will help ensure you receive all the nutrients necessary while altering your food habits. This is a fairly new movement in the wellness industry, but an incredibly impactful one. A comprehensive "Greens" supplement can work wonders for helping you stay energized, maintain healthy immune function, and maintain healthy alkalinity in the body; most illnesses cannot survive in a body with healthy alkalinity, so this is a big step towards better overall health that I enjoy taking on a daily basis, not only while cleansing.

I really adore Green Vibrance Plant-based Advanced Daily Superfood, hat also includes probiotics, alkalizing minerals, and a bundle of other amazing superfoods to help you along your way. I took one-half scoop two times daily, but more may be desired during Level 3 (when you are juicing) to maintain optimal immune function.

Kelp***: Kelp is another vastly underrated gem that helps speed up the metabolism by helping the thyroid and other glands by stimulating digestive secretions. This will help burn excess calories and ensure your food metabolizes quicker and it also does wonders for the skin, hair and nails, among other things. Healers of Ancient Greece used kelp in the treatment of thyroid disorders, arthritis, high blood pressure, colds, poor digestion, and a number of other ailments. Ancient Japanese texts allude to kelp being a powerful remedy for kidney, bladder, and prostate ailments, among other things, reserved only for nobility in those times.

Today, concentrated kelp in a variety of forms is still widely used in cancer treatments and for correcting issues related to thyroid malfunction, particularly hypothyroidism. It is an excellent source of iodine and helps boost metabolic functionality.

I really adore Green Vibrance Plant-based Advanced Daily Superfood (mentioned above), which also includes probiotics, alkalizing minerals, and a bundle of other amazing super-foods to help you along your way. I took one-half scoop two times daily during my cleanse and sometimes three times daily during Level 3.

Licorice Root*: Licorice Root was a favorite remedy of many ancient cultures including the Egyptians, the Babylonians, Hindus, and Romans, to name a few. The sought-after herb contains essential vitamins and minerals that help give energy to your system and also improves circulation while assisting with lung, blood, and bronchial cleansing. It was said to improve stamina, reduce appetite, and revitalize tired warriors before battle.

Licorice Root sometimes has an overpowering taste when taken in liquid form, a taste I personally find rather unpleasant. For that reason alone, there is enough for me in Nature's Secret – Super Cleanse Tablets (previously discussed), which includes Licorice Root and a number of other ingredients on this list, noted with one asterisk. I took one tablet three times daily, as directed, during my cleanse. Licorice Root in many forms is readily available.

Maca (Powder): I was first introduced to the wonders of Maca in Peru, where native Medicine Men recommend Maca for a number of thyroid and endocrine issues. Naturally this was one of the first things I asked about when researching in Peru. In ancient times, it was used to increase sexual stamina or fertility, and is still said to help improve the overall health of the reproductive and sexual organs, among other things. In mainstream herbal arenas, it is still marketed to promote higher energy levels and overall stamina. Maca is easily added to juices or meals and works quickly in powder form.

Though it can be grown in other regions of the world, Maca is significantly less potent when grown outside of the Andean mountains. The scarcity of truly high-quality Maca makes it a very special treat, and I simply cannot bring enough home when I travel to Peru.

When I purchase it in the US, lean towards Gaia Herbs Gelatanized Maca Powder and can rely on them to source high-quality Maca. I took one teaspoon twice daily mixed with water, when I took my greens powder and still enjoy taking it on a daily basis.

Probiotics: This is essential in maintaining healthy bacteria in the digestive system as well as regulating sugars and assisting with any sort of candida or yeast issues. While there may be some in whatever greens supplement you're taking, it's recommended you take additional probiotics to ensure you are getting plenty throughout this process, especially if you are incorporating more fruits into your diet.

Ancient Egyptians, particularly the nobility, were accustomed to consuming fermented milk products in order to treat stomach and intestinal ailments. Healers of later times discovered that fermentation, previously used only for preserving food, was a healthy tool for combatting a myriad of other issues like scurvy, and also strengthened immune function.

Hippocrates, the Father of Western Medicine, was famous for saying that "all disease begins in the gut." He was also a firm believer in the intestinal and digestive benefits of fermented milk as a medicine.

I love Garden of Life RAW Probiotics – Colon Care, which packs 50 billion active probiotics into one little capsule. The "Colon Care" variety seems appropriate for deep cleansing circumstances, but any live/raw probiotic can be quite effective. I took one tablet daily, mid-day, during my cleanse.

Psyllium Husks/Flakes: Ancient Ayurveda suggest using Psyllium as an antidiarrheal, and digestive detoxification agent. I discovered it is commonly used in the Middle East as a digestive cleansing agent, available in many traditional spice or grain markets.

Psyllium is a crucial part of the detox process and the high fiber content of psyllium also greatly assists in helping you feel "full" during Level 3.

When properly combined with liquid Bentonite clay, Psyllium becomes an even more powerful detox tool; this method I learned from Dr. Richard Anderson's cleansing regimens, and I highly recommend reading his books if you are interested in other methods of deep internal cleansing. When properly mixed, as described below, Psyllium will help bind toxins and flush them from your system quickly and effectively.

Organic is <u>very</u> important with psyllium due to the texture of the husks, which could easily store chemicals and pesticides if not organically grown. I like Organic India Whole Husk Psyllium, but many varieties are available. I took two tablespoons three times daily mixed with Bentonite and 10 oz of distilled water, as shown in the calendar. To be clear, unlike many of the ingredients listed, this detox mixture is *not* to be taken with other herbs and supplements.

Trace Minerals: Because high crop yields were so important to the ecosystem of the Mayan civilization, they were constantly researching ways to improve yields via various methods of their time. One significant improvement was the supplementation of minerals, via specialized fertilization. This concept was adopted by other civilizations throughout the Americas and evolved into the supplementation of trace minerals for humans to correct illnesses of the major organs, heart problems, glandular issues, and hormonal imbalances. Trace amounts of Iodine, calcium, Copper, silver and other minerals are vital to the human body and are rarely derived from food in this era.

With that in mind, we may not get the vitamins and minerals we need from our food or juice, so it's important to supplement these with quality trace minerals when eliminating solids from the diet. This will help ensure the body is functioning optimally throughout the entire deep cleansing process. Not only did these minerals help keep me going energetically, but they worked wonders for boosting my mood and raising energy levels throughout every Level of the cleanse.

I find that Source Naturals Colloidal Trace Minerals and Electrolytes to be a very effective formula. I took one full dropper three times daily during my cleanse.

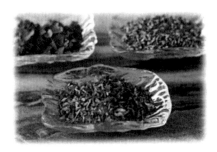

Chapter Sixteen
My Optional Ingredients

Barberry*: This often forgotten herb can help eliminate constipation while serving as an effective stomach, intestine, and colon cleanser.

I like Nature's Secret – Super Cleanse Tablets (previously mentioned), which includes this and a number of other ingredients on this list, noted with one asterisk. I took one tablet three times daily during my cleanse.

Echinacea**: Though typically an "active responder" for homeopathic medicine, this infamous immune-booster works wonders for helping the body ease into changes in diet and maintain healthy immune function while cleansing. If you are prone to illness and want to ensure you maintain great health throughout your cleanse, this is a great option and it often comes coupled with Goldenseal Root, which is a required ingredient.

I like Herb Pharm Echinacea Goldenseal compound extract (Goldenseal was mentioned already), which effectively combines both herbs in one formula, noted with two asterisks. Try to get the alcohol-free version, if possible. I took one full dropper three times daily, as directed, during my cleanse.

Fennel Seed*: Another great multitasker, Fennel helps remove impurities, aid in ridding the body of parasitic substances and is a superb appetite suppressant, among other things.

I like Nature's Secret – Super Cleanse Tablets (previously mentioned), which includes this and a number of other ingredients on this list, noted with one asterisk. I took one tablet three times daily during my cleanse.

Ginger Root*: Ginger is a marvelous superfood that helps relieve aches, pains and even gas, all while improving circulation and improving circulation.

Ginger root powder can be supplemented into your meals or juices.

For more controlled amounts, I like Nature's Secret – Super Cleanse Tablets (previously mentioned), which includes this and a number of other ingredients on this list, noted with one asterisk. I took one tablet three times daily during my cleanse.

Irish Moss*: This is a lesser-known secret weapon in helping to improve thyroid function. Irish moss has also been known to aid tumors, joint, and lung ailments in addition to improving intestinal functionality.

I like Nature's Secret – Super Cleanse Tablets (previously mentioned), which includes this and a number of other ingredients on this list, noted with one asterisk. I took one tablet three times daily during my cleanse.

Red Raspberry Leaf*: This helps improve digestion, eliminate wastes in the intestines, and stimulates the metabolic process in fantastic ways. It also supplies an excellent source of iron to the system and encourages healthy bowel movements while also preventing diarrhea. Raspberry ketones have similar effects, it's all very closely related if you're substituting one for another.

I like Nature's Secret – Super Cleanse Tablets (previously mentioned), which includes this and a number of other ingredients on this list, noted with one asterisk. I took one tablet three times daily.

Rose Hips: This is excellent for helping address issues related to stress, infections, cancers, cramps, colds, and a bevy of other ailments. Rose Hips are vitamin-rich and can be an excellent super-food when incorporated into a cleanse regimen.

I like Starwest Botanicals Organic Rosehips Powder, which can easily be added to your greens when you take those.

> **Note:** Be sure you choose an edible product as many Rose Hips products on the market are for external use. Amounts I used varied, but use as directed and feel free to mix it with greens.

Yellow Dock: This amazing source of iron has been known to aide in fighting free radicals, and incorporated into treatments for leukemia, cancers, and even leprosy. This stimulates elimination channels for the body (especially the skin and sweat glands), which is a superb booster to any deep cleanse recipe.

I like Herb Pharm Yellow Dock herbal extract. I took one fully dropper three times daily during my cleanse.

Chapter Seventeen
Amounts and Timing

Now that you know the What and Why, it's time to consider the How and When. This can seem like an overwhelming process, but it's not! I've simplified it all for you by laying out my routine. Once you have your ingredients together, refer back to this section to learn when I incorporated each item into my routine.

I've included a day planner for you to get a better idea of when I took what. You may be inspired by this and adjust it to suit your needs, please note the times in between each item must remain the same; for instance, do not take any supplements or herbs within two hours of consuming the psyllium and bentonite detox mixture as this mixture will inhibit their effectiveness. That being said, do not take any prescription medication three hours before or two hours after the detox mixture for the same reason.

VERY IMPORTANT NOTE:

Some items are meant to be taken on an empty stomach and this cleanse calendar (planner) was designed for optimal absorption, so it's best to adhere to the plan for ideal results.

**Do not consume anything two hours before OR one
hour following the Detox Mix (Water-Bentonite-
Psyllium Mixture).**

A customized planner for *The* Cleanse has been created for
you (one week planner for Level 1, one week planner for
Level 2, and one for Level 3). These three Planner pages are a
necessary part of the deep cleansing process, but they are
structured as calendars and were not legible here in this book.
They are waiting for you online at www.SupremelyBeing.com
/Planner where you may access them for free, any time, from
any device, and also download them in a number of formats.

Chapter Eighteen
Shopping List

There are a bevy of fantastic companies creating delicious raw food these days. Unprocessed, whole raw food is key to optimal cleansing, and also a sustainable approach to making incredible long-term changes. To learn about the delicious raw products on the market and to get relevant updates on health, cleanses, diet hacks, recipes, and living a more conscious lifestyle, please follow **@SupremelyBeing** on Twitter and Like us on Facebook **@SupremelyBeing**.

So, now that you have the low-down on what will be going into your body during this detox process, let me simplify things by filling you in on what to buy. Most of these items can be purchased from the same place.

My go-to spot is Vitacost.com (great prices and lightning fast shipping).

Bonus: New customers receive $10 off their first order using this link: http://goo.gl/EQ5Q5h (the VitaCost website).

Natural food grocers like Whole Foods, Jimbo's, and Sprouts may offer most, if not all, of the items, but the price may be a bit higher and selections may be limited. Alternatively, Amazon is a great place to shop, if you find trusted sellers (preferably with Amazon fulfillment), and you don't mind taking the extra time to shop around a little.

Thank You

Thank you to all of the Doctors, Shamans, Healers, Medicine Men, and tribespeople who dedicate their lives to wellness. Thank you to all who share their questions, thoughts, and experiences with the world; every relative book, every medical journal, every health blog, every forum post, and every motivational social media share adds fuel to the fire that is human wellness.

Thank you to all of the loving creators who have dedicated their culinary talents to putting whole, raw snacks and treats on the market – staying on track with a cleanse or raw diet is easier now than ever because of your innovative solutions!

Most importantly, thank *you* for reading this book. I am so grateful for your curiosity and wish you nothing but the happiest, healthiest times ahead on your journey... To our health!

Made in the USA
San Bernardino, CA
27 March 2017